# 39 Organic Juice Recipes to Clear Away Bad Breath:

## Eliminate Having Bad Breath and a Dry Mouth in a Matter of Days

By

**Joe Correa CSN**

## COPYRIGHT

© 2017 Live Stronger Faster Inc.

All rights reserved

Reproduction or translation of any part of this work beyond that permitted by section 107 or 108 of the 1976 United States Copyright Act without the permission of the copyright owner is unlawful.

This publication is designed to provide accurate and authoritative information in regard to the subject matter covered. It is sold with the understanding that neither the author nor the publisher is engaged in rendering medical advice. If medical advice or assistance is needed, consult with a doctor. This book is considered a guide and should not be used in any way detrimental to your health. Consult with a physician before starting this nutritional plan to make sure it's right for you.

## ACKNOWLEDGEMENTS

This book is dedicated to my friends and family that have had mild or serious illnesses so that you may find a solution and make the necessary changes in your life.

# 39 Organic Juice Recipes to Clear Away Bad Breath:

Eliminate Having Bad Breath and a Dry Mouth in a Matter of Days

By

**Joe Correa CSN**

## CONTENTS

Copyright

Acknowledgements

About The Author

Introduction

39 Organic Juice Recipes to Clear Away Bad Breath: Eliminate Having Bad Breath and a Dry Mouth in a Matter of Days

Additional Titles from This Author

## ABOUT THE AUTHOR

After years of Research, I honestly believe in the positive effects that proper nutrition can have over the body and mind. My knowledge and experience has helped me live healthier throughout the years and which I have shared with family and friends. The more you know about eating and drinking healthier, the sooner you will want to change your life and eating habits.

Nutrition is a key part in the process of being healthy and living longer so get started today. The first step is the most important and the most significant.

## INTRODUCTION

39 Organic Juice Recipes to Clear Away Bad Breath: Eliminate Having Bad Breath and a Dry Mouth in a Matter of Days

By Joe Correa CSN


Sometimes, even with the best possible oral hygiene, we can't seem to prevent bad breath. This can become extremely frustrating and affect our confidence in so many different ways. Unfortunately, bad breath is not always a reflection of our dental health. Bad breath can be related to different digestive problems and the overall state of our gastrointestinal tract. The best way to prevent and solve this problem is to take care of our entire digestive tract along with our teeth.

The key to a healthy and clean digestive tract and fresh breath lies in the food we eat. Just like with everything else in our body, food has the ability to do some serious damage as well as the ability to heal us. When we talk about bad breath, there are some specific foods we have to consume in order to clean our mouth and destroy the bacteria responsible for these problems. Apples, carrots, and celery are among the best foods to help you fight bad breath. Unsweetened black or green tea are also proven to help fight off bad breath. They contain some powerful antioxidants that help destroy the bacteria growing in your mouth and other parts of a digestive system. Parsley, ginger, and basil, on the other hand, have the ability to directly neutralize the effects of a heavy, garlic-based lunch. Some other, bad breath fighting foods are cherries, lettuce, and spinach.

I have used my extensive nutritional knowledge and experience to create a great collection of bad breath preventing juice recipes. These juices are based on the ingredients mentioned above and then combined with some other foods for a superb taste you will absolutely love. Take a few minutes every day to prepare yourself a healthy juice that will give you a cleaner and fresher breath naturally. You deserve it!

# 39 ORGANIC JUICE RECIPES TO CLEAR AWAY BAD BREATH: ELIMINATE HAVING BAD BREATH AND A DRY MOUTH IN A MATTER OF DAYS

1. **Strawberry Mint Juice**

**Ingredients:**

1 cup of strawberries, chopped

1 cup of fresh mint, torn

1 large Granny Smith's apple, cored and chopped

1 large banana, peeled

2 oz of water

**Preparation:**

Wash the strawberries and remove the stems. Cut into bite-sized pieces and fill the measuring cup. Reserve the rest in the refrigerator. Set aside.

Wash the mint thoroughly under cold running water. Drain and torn into small pieces. Set aside.

Wash the apple and cut lengthwise in half. Remove the core and chop into small pieces. Set aside.

Peel the banana and cut into small chunks. Set aside.

Now, combine strawberries, mint, apple, and banana in a juicer. Process until well juiced. Transfer to a serving glass and stir in the water.

Add some ice and serve immediately.

**Nutrition information per serving:** Kcal: 245, Protein: 4.3g, Carbs: 73.8g, Fats: 1.5g

## 2. Pomegranate Apple Juice

**Ingredients:**

1 cup of pomegranate seeds

1 medium-sized apple, cored

1 cup of mango, chunked

1 small ginger slice

¼ tsp of cinnamon, ground

1 oz of water

**Preparation:**

Cut the top of the pomegranate fruit using a sharp paring knife. Slice down to each of the white membranes inside of the fruit. Pop the seeds into a measuring cup and set aside.

Wash the apple and cut lengthwise in half. Remove the core and cut into small pieces. Set aside.

Peel the mango and cut into chunks. Fill the measuring cup and reserve the rest in the refrigerator. Set aside.

Peel the ginger slice and chop into small pieces. Set aside.

Now, combine pomegranate seeds, apple, mango, and ginger in a juicer and process until juiced. Transfer to a serving glass and stir in the cinnamon and water.

Refrigerate for 5 minutes before serving.

**Nutrition information per serving:** Kcal: 227, Protein: 3.6g, Carbs: 64.1g, Fats: 1.9g

## 3. Blueberry Lemon Juice

**Ingredients:**

1 cup of blueberries

1 whole lemon, halved

1 Golden Delicious apple, cored

1 whole kiwi, peeled and chopped

¼ tsp of ginger, ground

1 oz of water

**Preparation:**

Place the blueberries in a colander. Rinse well under cold running water and drain. Fill the measuring cup and reserve the rest in the refrigerator.

Peel the lemon and cut lengthwise in half. Set aside.

Wash the apple and cut lengthwise in half. Remove the core and cut into bite-sized pieces and set aside.

Peel the kiwi and cut into small pieces. Make sure to reserve the kiwi juice while cutting.

Now, combine blueberries, lemon, apple, and kiwi in a juicer and process until juiced. Transfer to a serving glass and stir in the ginger, water, and reserved kiwi juice.

Add some crushed ice and serve immediately.

**Nutrition information per serving:** Kcal: 217, Protein: 3.2g, Carbs: 66.2g, Fats: 1.3g

## 4. Raspberry Lime Juice

**Ingredients:**

1 cup of raspberries

1 whole lime, peeled

1 medium-sized Red Delicious apple, cored

1 whole plum, pitted and chopped

1 oz of water

**Preparation:**

Place the raspberries in a colander and rinse well under cold running water. Drain and fill the measuring cup. Reserve the rest in the refrigerator. Set aside.

Peel the lime and cut lengthwise in half. Cut into quarters and set aside.

Wash the apple and cut lengthwise in half. Remove the core and cut into bite-sized pieces. Set aside.

Wash the plum and cut in half. Remove the pit and chop into small pieces. Set aside.

Now, combine raspberries, lime, apple, and plum in a juicer and process until juiced. Transfer to a serving glass and stir in the water.

Refrigerate for 10 minutes before serving.

**Nutrition information per serving:** Kcal: 173, Protein: 2.7g, Carbs: 55.7g, Fats: 1.4g

## 5. Broccoli Fennel Juice

**Ingredients:**

2 cups of broccoli, chopped

1 cup of fennel, chopped

1 medium-sized Granny Smith's apple, cored

1 cup of fresh basil, chopped

1 oz of water

**Preparation:**

Wash the broccoli and trim off the outer leaves. Chop into small pieces and fill the measuring cup. Reserve the rest for later. Set aside.

Trim off the fennel stalks and outer wilted layers. Wash and chop the fennel into bite-sized pieces. Fill the measuring cup and reserve the rest for later. Set aside.

Wash the apple and cut lengthwise in half. Remove the core and chop into small pieces. Set aside.

Rinse the basil thoroughly under cold running water. Drain and torn into small pieces. Set aside.

Now, combine broccoli, fennel, apple, and basil in a juicer and process until juiced. Transfer to a serving glass and stir in the water.

Refrigerate for 10 minutes before serving.

**Nutrition information per serving:** Kcal: 140, Protein: 7.7g, Carbs: 41.8g, Fats: 1.3g

## 6. Cantaloupe Orange Juice

**Ingredients:**

1 cup of cantaloupe, chopped

1 large orange, peeled

1 cup of fresh mint, torn

1 cup of blackberries

¼ tsp of cinnamon, ground

**Preparation:**

Cut the cantaloupe in half. Scrape out the seeds and cut one large wedge. Peel and chop into small pieces. Fill the measuring cup and wrap the rest in a plastic foil. Refrigerate for later.

Peel the orange and divide into wedges. Cut each wedge in half and set aside.

Rinse the mint under cold running water and drain. Torn into small pieces and set aside.

Place the blackberries in a colander and rinse well. Drain and set aside.

Now, combine cantaloupe, orange, mint, and blackberries in a juicer and process until juiced. Transfer to a serving glass and stir in the cinnamon.

Add some ice and serve immediately.

**Nutrition information per serving:** Kcal: 157, Protein: 5.9g, Carbs: 51.9g, Fats: 1.5g

## 7. Pumpkin Lemon Juice

**Ingredients:**

1 cup of pumpkin, cubed

1 small Golden Delicious apple, cored and chopped

1 whole lemon, peeled and halved

1 large carrot, sliced

1 cup of watercress, torn

**Preparation:**

Cut the top of a pumpkin. Cut lengthwise in half and then scrape out the seeds. Cut one large wedge and peel it. Cut into small cubes and fill the measuring cup. Reserve the rest in the refrigerator.

Wash the apple and cut lengthwise in half. Remove the core and cut into bite-sized pieces. Set aside.

Peel the lemon and cut lengthwise in half. Set aside.

Wash and peel the carrot. Cut into thin slices and set aside.

Rinse the watercress thoroughly under cold running water. Drain and torn into small pieces. Set aside.

Now, combine pumpkin, apple, lemon, carrot, and watercress in a juicer and process until juiced. Transfer to a serving glass and add some ice before serving.

Enjoy!

**Nutrition information per serving:** Kcal: 126, Protein: 3.6g, Carbs: 37.8g, Fats: 0.7g

## 8. Mango Strawberry Juice

**Ingredients:**

1 whole mango, chopped

1 cup of strawberries, chopped

1 whole lime, peeled

1 large pear, chopped

1 cup of fresh mint, torn

1 tbsp of coconut water

**Preparation:**

Peel the mango and chop into small chunks or cubes. Set aside.

Wash the strawberries and remove the stems. Cut into bite-sized pieces and fill the measuring cup. Reserve the rest in the refrigerator.

Peel the lime and cut lengthwise in half. Set aside.

Wash the pear and cut in half. Remove the core and chop into small pieces. Set aside.

Rinse the mint thoroughly under cold running water and drain. Torn into small pieces and set aside.

Now, combine mango, strawberries, lime, pear, and mint in a juicer and process until juiced. Transfer to serving glass and stir in the coconut water.

Add some crushed ice and serve immediately.

**Nutrition information per serving:** Kcal: 335, Protein: 5.7g, Carbs: 103g, Fats: 2.3g

## 9. Grapefruit Apple Juice

**Ingredients:**

1 whole grapefruit, peeled and wedged

1 medium-sized apple, cored

3 whole apricots, pitted

1 cup of Swiss chard, torn

1 tbsp of liquid honey

¼ tsp of ginger, ground

**Preparation:**

Peel the grapefruit and divide into wedges. Cut each wedge in half and set aside.

Wash the apple and cut lengthwise in half. Remove the core and chop into bite-sized pieces. Set aside.

Wash the apricots and cut into halves. Chop all into small pieces and set aside.

Rinse the Swiss chard thoroughly under cold running water. Drain and torn into small pieces. Set aside.

Now, combine grapefruit, apple, apricots, and Swiss chard in a juicer and process until juiced. Transfer to a serving glass and stir in the honey and ginger.

Add few ice cubes and serve immediately.

**Nutrition information per serving:** Kcal: 212, Protein: 4.7g, Carbs: 61.9g, Fats: 1.1g

## 10. Cherry Pineapple Juice

**Ingredients:**

1 cup of cherries, pitted

1 cup of pineapple, chunked

1 cup of spinach, chopped

1 whole lemon, peeled

¼ tsp of cinnamon, ground

1 oz of water

**Preparation:**

Place the cherries in a medium colander. Rinse well under cold running water and remove the stems, if any. Cut each in half and remove the pits. Fill the measuring cup and reserve the rest in the refrigerator.

Using a sharp paring knife, cut the top of the pineapple. Gently remove all hard skin and slice it into thin slices. Fill the measuring cup and reserve the rest for later.

Rinse the spinach thoroughly under cold running water. Drain and chop into small pieces. Set aside.

Peel the lemon and cut lengthwise in half. Set aside.

Now, combine cherries, pineapple, spinach, and lemon in a juicer and process until juiced. Transfer to a serving glass and stir in the water.

Add some crushed ice and serve immediately.

**Nutrition information per serving:** Kcal: 196, Protein: 9.2g, Carbs: 59.3g, Fats: 1.5g

## 11. Tomato Parsley Juice

**Ingredients:**

2 medium-sized Roma tomatoes, chopped

1 cup of fresh parsley, torn

1 medium-sized artichoke, chopped

1 cup of Romaine lettuce, torn

¼ tsp of salt

¼ tsp of dried oregano, ground

**Preparation:**

Wash the tomatoes and place in a bowl. Chop into small pieces and make sure to reserve the tomato juice while cutting. Set aside.

Combine parsley and lettuce in a large colander. Rinse well under cold running water and drain. Torn into small pieces and set aside.

Wash the artichoke trim off the outer leaves. Chop into bite-sized pieces and fill the measuring cup. Reserve the rest in the refrigerator. Set aside.

Now, combine tomatoes, parsley, artichoke, and lettuce in a juicer and process until juiced. Transfer to a serving glass and stir in the salt and oregano.

Refrigerate for 10 minutes before serving.

Enjoy!

**Nutrition information per serving:** Kcal: 82, Protein: 8.7g, Carbs: 28.3g, Fats: 1.3g

## 12. Avocado Beet Juice

**Ingredients:**

1 cup of avocado, cubed

1 cup of beets, sliced

1 cup of celery, cut into bite-sized pieces

1 whole lemon, peeled

1 oz of water

**Preparation:**

Peel the avocado and cut lengthwise in half. Remove the pit and cut into small cubes. Fill the measuring cup and reserve the rest in the refrigerator. Set aside.

Wash the beets and trim off the green ends. Slightly peel and cut into thin slices. Fill the measuring cup and reserve the rest for later.

Wash the celery and cut into bite-sized pieces. Fill the measuring cup and reserve the rest in the refrigerator.

Peel the lemon and cut lengthwise in half. Set aside.

Now, combine avocado, beets, celery, and lemon in a juicer. Process until juiced.

Transfer to a serving glass and stir in the water. Refrigerate for 10 minutes before serving.

**Nutrition information per serving:** Kcal: 264, Protein: 6.5g, Carbs: 34.2g, Fats: 22.5g

## 13. Papaya Orange Juice

**Ingredients:**

1 cup of papaya, chopped

1 large orange, peeled

1 small Granny Smith's apple, cored

1 cup of fresh mint, torn

1 tbsp of fresh basil, torn

**Preparation:**

Wash and peel the papaya. Cut lengthwise in half and scoop out the seeds. Cut into bite-sized pieces and fill the measuring cup. Reserve the rest in the refrigerator.

Peel the orange and divide into wedges. Cut each wedge in half and set aside.

Wash the apple and cut in half. Remove the core and cut into bite-sized pieces. Set aside.

Rinse the mint and basil thoroughly under cold running water. Drain and torn into small pieces. Set aside.

Now, combine papaya, orange, apple, mint, and basil in a juicer and process until juiced. Transfer to a serving glass and add some ice.

Serve immediately.

**Nutrition information per serving:** Kcal: 199, Protein: 4.1g, Carbs: 60.1g, Fats: 1.1g

## 14. Cabbage Zucchini Juice

**Ingredients:**

1 cup of purple cabbage, torn

1 medium-sized zucchini, sliced

1 cup of celery, chopped

1 cup of cucumber, sliced

¼ tsp of ginger, ground

¼ tsp of turmeric, ground

¼ tsp of salt

**Preparation:**

Rinse the purple cabbage under cold running water. Drain and torn into small pieces and set aside.

Wash the zucchini and cut into thin slices. Set aside.

Wash the celery and chop into bite-sized pieces. Set aside.

Wash the cucumber and cut into slices. Fill the measuring cup and reserve the rest for later.

Now, combine cabbage, zucchini, celery, and cucumber in a juicer and process until juiced. Transfer to a serving glass and stir in the ginger, turmeric, and salt.

Refrigerate for 10 minutes before serving.

**Nutrition information per serving:** Kcal: 62, Protein: 4.7g, Carbs: 17.5g, Fats: 1g

## 15. Strawberry Squash Juice

**Ingredients:**

1 cup of strawberries, chopped

1 cup of butternut squash, cubed

2 whole plums, pitted and chopped

1 medium-sized apple, cored

¼ tsp of ginger, ground

¼ tsp of turmeric, ground

**Preparation:**

Wash the strawberries and remove the stems. Cut into bite-sized pieces and fill the measuring cup. Reserve the rest in the refrigerator. Set aside.

Peel the butternut squash and cut lengthwise in half. Scoop out the seeds and wash the both halves. Cut into small cubes and fill the measuring cup. Wrap the rest of the squash in a plastic foil and refrigerate for later.

Wash the plums and cut in half. Remove the pits and cut into bite-sized pieces. Set aside.

Wash the apple and cut lengthwise in half. Remove the core and cut into bite-sized pieces. Set aside.

Now, combine strawberries, butternut squash, plum, and apple in a juicer and process until well juiced. Transfer to a serving glass and add some crushed ice.

Serve immediately.

**Nutrition information per serving:** Kcal: 214, Protein: 4.1g, Carbs: 65.2g, Fats: 1.2g

## 16. Cauliflower Parsnip Juice

**Ingredients:**

1 cup of cauliflower, chopped

1 cup of parsnip, sliced

1 large carrot, sliced

1 cup of fennel, trimmed and chopped

1 whole lime, peeled

**Preparation:**

Wash the cauliflower and trim off the outer leaves. Cut into small pieces and fill the measuring cup. Reserve the rest for later.

Wash and peel the parsnip. Cut into thin slices and fill the measuring cup. Reserve the rest for later.

Trim off the fennel stalks and outer wilted layers. Wash and chop the fennel into bite-sized pieces. Fill the measuring cup and reserve the rest for later. Set aside.

Peel the lime and cut lengthwise in half. Set aside.

Now, combine cauliflower, parsnip, carrot, fennel, and lime in a juicer. Process until well juiced.

Transfer to a serving glass and refrigerate for 10 minutes before serving.

Add some turmeric or ginger for some extra taste. However, it's optional.

**Nutrition information per serving:** Kcal: 141, Protein: 5.6g, Carbs: 46.2g, Fats: 1.1g

## 17. Orange Pear Juice

**Ingredients:**

1 medium-sized orange, peeled

1 medium-sized pear, chopped

1 cup of beets, chopped

1 small Golden Delicious apple, chopped

¼ tsp of cinnamon, ground

¼ tsp of ginger, ground

**Preparation:**

Peel the orange and divide into wedges. Cut each wedge in half and set aside.

Wash the pear and cut in half. Remove the core and chop into small pieces. Set aside.

Wash the beets and trim off the green ends. Cut into slices and fill the measuring cup. Reserve the rest for later.

Wash the apple and cut lengthwise in half. Remove the core and cut into bite-sized pieces. Set aside.

Now, combine orange, pear, beets, and apple in a juicer and process until juiced.

Transfer to a serving glass and stir in the cinnamon and ginger. Add some ice before serving.

Enjoy!

**Nutrition information per serving:** Kcal: 234, Protein: 4.4g, Carbs: 73.1g, Fats: 0.8g

## 18. Blueberry Grape Juice

**Ingredients:**

2 cups of blueberries

1 cup of black grapes

1 cup of fresh mint, torn

1 large banana, peeled

2 tbsp of milk

¼ tsp of cinnamon, ground

**Preparation:**

Place the blueberries in a colander. Rinse well under cold running water and drain. Set aside.

Wash the grapes and remove the stems. Fill the measuring cup and reserve the rest in the refrigerator. Set aside.

Wash the mint thoroughly under cold running water. Drain and torn into small pieces. Set aside.

Now, combine blueberries, grapes, mint, and banana in a juicer and process until juiced. Transfer to a serving glass and stir in the milk and cinnamon.

Refrigerate for 10 minutes before serving.

**Nutrition information per serving:** Kcal: 326, Protein: 6.2g, Carbs: 93.4g, Fats: 2.1g

## 19. Crookneck Squash Juice

**Ingredients:**

1 cup of crookneck squash, cubed

1 large orange, peeled

1 large carrot, sliced

1 whole lemon, peeled

1 cup of cucumber, sliced

¼ tsp of turmeric, ground

**Preparation:**

Wash the squash and chop into small cubes. Fill the measuring cup and reserve the rest in the refrigerator. Set aside.

Peel the orange and divide into wedges. Cut each wedge in half and set aside.

Wash and peel the carrot. Cut into thin slices and set aside.

Peel the lemon and cut lengthwise in half. Set aside.

Wash the cucumber and cut into thin slices. Fill the measuring cup and reserve the rest for later.

Now, combine squash, orange, carrot, lemon, and cucumber in a juicer and process until juiced. Transfer to a serving glass and stir in the turmeric.

Add some crushed ice and serve immediately.

**Nutrition information per serving:** Kcal: 127, Protein: 4.6g, Carbs: 40.7g, Fats: 0.9g

## 20. Kale Beet Juice

**Ingredients:**

1 cup of fresh kale, torn

1 cup of beets, sliced

1 small Granny Smith's apple, cored

1 cup of cantaloupe, cubed

¼ tsp of ginger, ground

**Preparation:**

Rinse the kale thoroughly under cold running water. Drain and torn into small pieces. Set aside.

Wash the beets and trim off the green ends. Cut into thin slices and fill the measuring cup. Reserve the rest for some other juice.

Wash the apple and cut lengthwise in half. Remove the core and cut into bite-sized pieces. Set aside.

Cut the cantaloupe in half. Scrape out the seeds and cut one large wedge. Peel and chop into small pieces. Fill the measuring cup and wrap the rest in a plastic foil. Refrigerate for later.

Now, combine kale, beets, apple, and cantaloupe in a juicer and process until juiced. Transfer to a serving glass and stir in the ginger.

Add some ice and serve immediately.

**Nutrition information per serving:** Kcal: 181, Protein: 7g, Carbs: 51.1g, Fats: 1.4g

## 21. Kiwi Mint Juice

**Ingredients:**

2 whole kiwis, peeled

1 cup of fresh mint, torn

1 cup of cucumber, sliced

1 medium-sized Golden Delicious apple, cored

1 large banana, peeled

**Preparation:**

Peel the kiwis and cut lengthwise in half. Set aside.

Rinse the mint thoroughly under cold running water and drain. Torn into small pieces and set aside.

Wash the cucumber and cut into thin slices. Fill the measuring cup and reserve the rest for later. Set aside.

Wash the apple and cut lengthwise in half. Remove the core and cut into bite-sized pieces. Set aside.

Peel the banana and cut into thin slices. Set aside.

Now, combine kiwis, cucumber, apple, and banana in a juicer and process until juiced. Transfer to a serving glass and add some ice.

Serve immediately.

**Nutrition information per serving:** Kcal: 272, Protein: 4.8g, Carbs: 79.8g, Fats: 1.7g

## 22. Blackberry Mango Juice

**Ingredients:**

1 cup of blackberries

1 cup of mango, chunked

3 whole apricots, chopped

1 cup of fresh spinach, torn

1 whole lime, peeled

**Preparation:**

Rinse the blackberries using a large colander. Drain and set aside.

Peel the mango and cut into small chunks. Fill the measuring cup and reserve the rest for later. Set aside.

Wash the apricots and cut in half. Remove the pits and chop into small pieces. Set aside.

Rinse the spinach thoroughly under cold running water. Drain and torn into small pieces. Set aside.

Peel the lime and cut lengthwise in half. Set aside.

Now, combine blackberries, mango, apricots, spinach, and lime in a juicer. Process until juiced. Transfer to a serving glass and refrigerate for 10 minutes before serving.

Enjoy!

**Nutrition information per serving:** Kcal: 201, Protein: 11.1g, Carbs: 61.5g, Fats: 2.6g

## 23. Cranberry Peppermint Juice

**Ingredients:**

1 cup of cranberries

3 whole apricots, pitted and chopped

1 small Golden Delicious apple, cored

1 cup of cherries, pitted

1 tsp of peppermint extract

3 tbsp of coconut water

**Preparation:**

Rinse the cranberries using a large colander. Drain and set aside.

Wash the apricots and cut in half. Remove the pits and chop into small pieces. Set aside.

Wash the apple and cut lengthwise in half. Remove the core and chop into small pieces. Set aside.

Rinse the cherries under cold running water. Drain and cut each cherry in half. Remove the pits and set aside.

Now, combine cranberries, apricots, apple, and cherries in a juicer and process until juiced. Transfer to a serving glass and stir in the peppermint extract and coconut water.

Sprinkle with some finely chopped mint for some extra taste. However, it's optional.

Add few ice cubes and serve immediately.

**Nutrition information per serving:** Kcal: 216, Protein: 3.8g, Carbs: 66.1g, Fats: 1.1g

## 24.  Parsley Cucumber Juice

**Ingredients:**

2 cups of parsley, torn

1 whole cucumber, sliced

1 cup of celery, chopped

1 whole leek, chopped

1 cup of beet greens, torn

¼ tsp of turmeric powder, ground

¼ tsp of cumin, ground

**Preparation:**

Combine parsley and beet greens in a large colander. Rinse well under cold running water and drain. Torn into small pieces and set aside.

Wash the cucumber and cut into thin slices. Set aside.

Wash the celery and chop into small pieces. Fill the measuring cup and reserve the rest in the refrigerator. Set aside.

Wash the leek and chop into bite-sized pieces. Set aside.

Now, combine parsley, beet greens, cucumber, celery, and leek in a juicer and process until juiced. Transfer to a serving glass and stir in the turmeric and cumin.

Serve immediately.

**Nutrition information per serving:** Kcal: 127, Protein: 8.4g, Carbs: 35.7g, Fats: 1.7g

## 25.   Honeydew Melon-Swiss Chard Juice

**Ingredients:**

1 large wedge of honeydew melon, peeled and cubed

1 cup of Swiss chard, torn

1 large carrot, peeled and sliced

1 cup of cucumber, sliced

1 small ginger knob, peeled

¼ tsp of turmeric, ground

2 oz of water

**Preparation:**

Cut melon lengthwise in half. Scoop out the seeds and then wash. Cut one large wedge and peel it. Cut into small cubes and set aside.

Rinse the Swiss chard thoroughly under cold running water. Drain and torn into small pieces. Set aside.

Wash and peel the carrot. Cut into thin slices and set aside.

Wash the cucumber and cut into thin slices. Fill the measuring cup and reserve the rest for later. Set aside.

Peel the ginger knob and cut into small pieces. Set aside.

Now, combine melon, Swiss chard, carrot, and cucumber in a juicer and process until juiced. Transfer to a serving glass and stir in the turmeric and water.

Refrigerate for 10 minutes before serving.

**Nutrition information per serving:** Kcal: 92, Protein: 2.6g, Carbs: 25.7g, Fats: 0.5g

## 26.  Celery Apple Juice

**Ingredients:**

1 cup of celery, chopped

1 large Granny Smith's apple, cored and chopped

1 small ginger knob, peeled

1 cup of fresh mint, torn

¼ tsp of liquid honey

1 oz of water

**Preparation:**

Wash the celery and chop into small pieces. Fill the measuring cup and reserve the rest for later.

Wash the apple and cut lengthwise in half. Remove the core and cut into bite-sized pieces. Set aside.

Peel the ginger knob and chop into small pieces. Set aside.

Rinse the mint thoroughly under cold running water. Dran and torn into small pieces.

Now, combine celery, apple, ginger, and mint in a juicer and process until well juiced. Transfer to a serving glass and stir in the honey and water.

Refrigerate for 10 minutes before serving.

Enjoy!

**Nutrition information per serving:** Kcal: 121, Protein: 2.6g, Carbs: 35.8g, Fats: 0.8g

## 27. Plum Pomegranate Juice

**Ingredients:**

3 whole plums, pitted and chopped

1 cup of pomegranate seeds

1 cup of pumpkin, cubed

1 medium-sized orange, peeled

¼ tsp of ginger, ground

1 oz of water

**Preparation:**

Wash the plums and cut into halves. Remove the pits and chop into small pieces. Set aside.

Cut the top of the pomegranate fruit using a sharp paring knife. Slice down to each of the white membranes inside of the fruit. Pop the seeds into a measuring cup and set aside.

Cut the top of a pumpkin. Cut lengthwise in half and then scrape out the seeds. Cut one large wedge and peel it. Cut into small cubes and fill the measuring cup. Reserve the rest in the refrigerator.

Peel the orange and divide into wedges. Cut each wedge in half and set aside.

Now, combine plums, pomegranate, pumpkin, and orange in a juicer. Process until juiced. Transfer to a serving glass and stir in the ginger and water.

Refrigerate for 10 minutes before serving.

Enjoy!

**Nutrition information per serving:** Kcal: 214, Protein: 5.2g, Carbs: 61.8g, Fats: 1.8g

## 28. Pepper Fennel Juice

**Ingredients:**

2 large red bell peppers, seeds removed

1 cup of fennel, trimmed and chopped

1 cup of spinach, torn

1 cup of cucumber, sliced

¼ tsp of salt

¼ tsp of cayenne pepper, ground

**Preparation:**

Wash the bell peppers and cut each lengthwise in half. Remove the stem and seeds. Chop into small pieces and set aside.

Trim off the fennel stalks and outer wilted layers. Wash and chop the fennel into bite-sized pieces. Fill the measuring cup and reserve the rest for later. Set aside.

Rinse the spinach thoroughly under cold running water. Drain and torn into small pieces. Fill the measuring cup and reserve the rest in the refrigerator.

Wash the cucumber and cut into thin slices. Fill the measuring cup and reserve the rest for later.

Now, combine bell peppers, fennel, spinach, and cucumber in a juicer and process until juiced. Transfer to a serving glass and stir in the salt and cayenne pepper.

Serve cold.

**Nutrition information per serving:** Kcal: 125, Protein: 10.6g, Carbs: 35.65g, Fats: 2.1g

## 29. Peach Apple Juice

**Ingredients:**

1 large peach, pitted

1 medium-sized Granny Smith's apple, cored

1 whole lemon, peeled

1 cup of mango, chunked

¼ tsp of cinnamon, ground

**Preparation:**

Wash the peach and cut in half. Remove the pit and chop into small pieces. Set aside.

Wash the apple and cut lengthwise in half. Remove the core and chop into bite-sized pieces. Set aside.

Peel the lemon and cut lengthwise in half. Set aside.

Peel the mango and cut into small chunks. Fill the measuring cup and reserve the rest in the refrigerator. Set aside.

Now, combine peach, apple, lemon, and mango in a juicer and process until juiced. Transfer to a serving glass and stir in the cinnamon.

Add some crushed ice and serve immediately.

Enjoy!

**Nutrition information per serving:** Kcal: 236, Protein: 4.3g, Carbs: 69.5g, Fats: 1.5g

## 30. Avocado Blueberry Juice

**Ingredients:**

1 cup of avocado, cubed

1 cup of blueberries

1 whole grapefruit, peeled

1 small Red Delicious apple, cored

1 tsp of peppermint extract

**Preparation:**

Peel the avocado and cut lengthwise in half. Remove the pit and cut into small cubes. Fill the measuring cup and reserve the rest in the refrigerator.

Place the blueberries in a colander. Rinse well under cold running water and drain. Set aside.

Peel the grapefruit and divide into wedges. Cut each wedge in half and set aside.

Wash the apple and cut lengthwise in half. Remove the core and cut into bite-sized pieces. Set aside.

Now, combine avocado, blueberries, grapefruit, and apple in a juicer and process until juiced. Transfer to a serving glass and stir in the peppermint extract. Refrigerate for 15 minutes before serving.

**Nutrition information per serving:** Kcal: 436, Protein: 6.4g, Carbs: 69.5g, Fats: 23.2g

## 31.  Strawberry Lemon Juice

**Ingredients:**

1 cup of strawberries, chopped

1 whole lemon, peeled

1 large banana, chunked

1 cup of pineapple, chunked

1 tbsp of fresh mint, finely chopped

**Preparation:**

Wash the strawberries and remove the stems. Chop into small pieces and fill the measuring cup. Reserve the rest in the refrigerator.

Peel the lemon and cut lengthwise in half. Set aside.

Peel the banana and cut into small chunks. Set aside.

Cut the top of the pineapple using a sharp paring knife. Gently remove all hard skin and slice it into thin slices. Fill the measuring cup and reserve the rest for later.

Now, combine strawberries, lemon, banana, and pineapple in a juicer. Process until juiced. Transfer to a serving glass and stir in the mint.

Add few ice cubes and serve immediately.

**Nutrition information per serving:** Kcal: 224, Protein: 4.1g, Carbs: 69.4g, Fats: 1.3g

## 32. Watermelon Celery Juice

**Ingredients:**

1 cup of watermelon, diced

1 cup of celery, chopped

1 cup of cherries, pitted

1 small ginger knob, peeled

1 oz of water

¼ tsp of cinnamon, ground

**Preparation:**

Cut the watermelon in half. Cut one large wedge and wrap the rest in a plastic foil and refrigerate. Dice the wedge and remove the pits. Fill the measuring cup and set aside.

Wash the celery and cut into small pieces. Fill the measuring cup and reserve the rest for later. Set aside.

Rinse the cherries under cold running water using a colander. Drain and cut each in half. Remove the pits and set aside.

Peel the ginger knob and cut into small pieces. Set aside.

Now, combine watermelon, celery, cherries, and ginger knob in a juicer and process until juiced. Transfer to a serving glass and stir in the water and cinnamon. Add some ice and serve immediately.

**Nutrition information per serving:** Kcal: 143, Protein: 3.4g, Carbs: 40.2g, Fats: 0.7g

## 33. Lettuce Tomato Juice

**Ingredients:**

2 cups of Romaine lettuce, chopped

1 medium-sized Roma tomato, chopped

1 cup of mustard greens, torn

1 cup of parsley, torn

1 whole cucumber, sliced

¼ tsp of turmeric, ground

¼ tsp of salt

**Preparation:**

Rinse the lettuce thoroughly under cold running water. Chop into small pieces and set aside.

Wash the tomato and place in a bowl. Chop into bite-sized pieces and reserve the tomato juice while cutting. Set aside.

Combine mustard greens and parsley in a large colander. Rinse well and drain. Torn into small pieces and set aside.

Wash the cucumber and cut into thin slices. Set aside.

Now, combine lettuce, tomato, mustard greens, parsley, and cucumber in a juicer and process until juiced. Transfer to a serving glass and stir in the turmeric, salt, and reserved tomato juice.

Refrigerate for 10 minutes before serving.

Enjoy!

**Nutrition information per serving:** Kcal: 85, Protein: 7.6g, Carbs: 25.3g, Fats: 1.6g

## 34. Potato Artichoke Juice

**Ingredients:**

1 cup of sweet potatoes, cubed

1 medium-sized artichoke, chopped

1 small zucchini, sliced

1 whole lime, peeled

1 large carrot, sliced

¼ tsp of salt

¼ tsp of turmeric, ground

**Preparation:**

Peel the potatoes and cut into small cubes. Place in a deep pot and add 3 cups of water. Bring it to a boil and cook for 5 minutes. Remove from the heat and drain well. Set aside to cool completely.

Wash the artichoke and trim off the outer leaves. Cut into small pieces and fill the measuring cup. Reserve the rest in the refrigerator.

Peel the zucchini and cut into thin slices. Set aside.

Peel the lime and cut lengthwise in half. Set aside.

Wash and peel the carrot. Cut into thin slices and set aside.

Now, combine potatoes, artichoke, zucchini, lime, and carrots in a juicer and process until juiced. Transfer to a serving glass and stir in the salt and turmeric.

Refrigerate for 10 minutes before serving.

**Nutrition information per serving:** Kcal: 177, Protein: 8.6g, Carbs: 54.5g, Fats: 0.8g

## 35. Cantaloupe Cranberry Juice

**Ingredients:**

1 cup of cantaloupe, diced

1 cup of cranberries

1 cup of blackberries

1 small Golden Delicious apple, cored

¼ tsp of cinnamon, ground

¼ tsp of ginger, ground

**Preparation:**

Cut the cantaloupe in half. Scrape out the seeds and cut one large wedge. Peel and dice into small pieces. Fill the measuring cup and wrap the rest in a plastic foil. Refrigerate for later.

Combine cranberries and blackberries in a large colander. Rinse well under cold running water and drain. Set aside.

Wash the apple cut lengthwise in half. Remove the core and cut into bite-sized pieces. Set aside.

Now, combine cantaloupe, cranberries, blackberries, and apple in a juicer and process until well juiced. Transfer to a serving glass and stir in the cinnamon and ginger.

Add some crushed ice and serve immediately.

Enjoy!

**Nutrition information per serving:** Kcal: 169, Protein: 4.1g, Carbs: 56.3g, Fats: 1.3g

## 36. Apricot Honey Juice

**Ingredients:**

1 cup of apricots, pitted and halved

1 tbsp of liquid honey

1 small Granny Smith's apple, cored

1 small pear, chopped

1 whole lemon, peeled and halved

1 cup of fresh mint, torn

**Preparation:**

Wash the apricots and cut each lengthwise in half. Remove the pits and fill the measuring cup. Reserve the rest in the refrigerator for some other juice.

Wash the apple and cut lengthwise in half. Remove the core and chop into bite-sized pieces. Set aside.

Wash the pear and cut in half. Remove the core and cut into small pieces. Set aside.

Peel the lemon and cut lengthwise in half. Set aside.

Rinse the mint thoroughly under cold running water. Drain and torn into small pieces. Set aside.

Now, combine apricots, apple, pear, lemon, and mint in a juicer and process until well juiced. Transfer to a serving glass and add some ice before serving.

Enjoy!

**Nutrition information per serving:** Kcal: 217, Protein: 4.9g, Carbs: 68.5g, Fats: 1.5g

## 37. Fennel Spinach Juice

**Ingredients:**

1 cup of fennel, chopped

1 cup of spinach, torn

1 cup of broccoli, chopped

1 whole lemon, peeled

1 whole lime, peeled

¼ tsp of ginger, ground

**Preparation:**

Trim off the fennel stalks and outer wilted layers. Wash and chop the fennel into bite-sized pieces. Fill the measuring cup and reserve the rest for later. Set aside.

Rinse the spinach thoroughly under cold running water and drain. Torn into small pieces and set aside.

Wash the broccoli and trim off the outer leaves. Chop into small pieces and fill the measuring cup. Reserve the rest in the refrigerator.

Peel the lemon and lime. Cut lengthwise into halves. Set aside.

Now, combine fennel, spinach, broccoli, lemon, and lime in a juicer. Process until juiced.

Transfer to a serving glass and stir in the ginger.

Add some crushed ice and serve immediately.

**Nutrition information per serving:** Kcal: 86, Protein: 10.5g, Carbs: 29.1g, Fats: 1.5g

## 38. Blueberry Vanilla Juice

**Ingredients:**

2 cups of blueberries

1 large wedge of honeydew melon

1 small Grany Smith's apple, cored

1 oz of coconut water

1 tsp of vanilla extract

1 tbsp of mint, finely chopped

**Preparation:**

Place the blueberries in a large colander. Rinse well under cold running water and drain. Set aside.

Cut melon lengthwise in half. Scoop out the seeds and then wash. Cut one large wedge and peel it. Cut into small cubes and set aside.

Wash the apple and cut lengthwise in half. Remove the core and cut into bite-sized pieces. Set aside.

Now, combine blueberries, honeydew melon, and apple in a juicer. Process until juiced.

Transfer to a serving glass and stir in the coconut water, vanilla extract, and mint. Add some crushed ice and serve immediately.

**Nutrition information per serving:** Kcal: 263, Protein: 3.7g, Carbs: 77.1g, Fats: 1.5g

## 39. Carrot Lime Juice

**Ingredients:**

1 large carrot, sliced

1 whole lime, peeled

1 cup of mango, chunked

1 large banana, sliced

1 small Golden Delicious apple, cored

¼ tsp of cinnamon, ground

**Preparation:**

Wash and peel the carrot. Cut into thin slices and set aside.

Peel the lime and cut lengthwise in half. Set aside.

Peel the mango and cut into small chunks. Fill the measuring cup and reserve the rest in the refrigerator. Set aside.

Peel the banana and cut into slices. Set aside.

Wash the apple and cut in half. Remove the core and chop into bite-sized pieces. Set aside.

Now, combine carrot, lime, mango, banana, and apple in a juicer and process until juiced. Transfer to a serving glass and stir in the cinnamon.

Add some ice and serve immediately.

**Nutrition information per serving:** Kcal: 290, Protein: 4.1g, Carbs: 83.9g, Fats: 1.5g

## ADDITIONAL TITLES FROM THIS AUTHOR

70 Effective Meal Recipes to Prevent and Solve Being Overweight: Burn Fat Fast by Using Proper Dieting and Smart Nutrition

By

Joe Correa CSN


48 Acne Solving Meal Recipes: The Fast and Natural Path to Fixing Your Acne Problems in Less Than 10 Days!

By

Joe Correa CSN


41 Alzheimer's Preventing Meal Recipes: Reduce or Eliminate Your Alzheimer's Condition in 30 Days or Less!

By

Joe Correa CSN


70 Effective Breast Cancer Meal Recipes: Prevent and Fight Breast Cancer with Smart Nutrition and Powerful Foods

By

Joe Correa CSN

www.ingramcontent.com/pod-product-compliance
Lightning Source LLC
Chambersburg PA
CBHW030301030426
42336CB00009B/474